Thank you for purchasing your new 21 Day I Love My Skin Journal. You are making the necessary steps to love all of you and keep your skin healthy!

In 21 days you will learn to love your skin and appreciate every aspect of your uniqueness.

Each day take time to read each affirmation, write about how your skin feels, and document any breakouts, flares, dryness, etc.

The goal is to
- Pinpoint your flares
- Notice how diet, stress, and emotions affects the skin
- To meet the goals you make for your skin.

I love you. Don't let insecurities or the photoshopped celebrities make you feel less than or love your skin any less.

Empresse

Write a letter to yourself about how your skin journey has impacted you, how it makes you feel, and what you hope to gain from this 21 day journey.

Dear _____

_____

_____

_____

_____

_____

_____

_____

_____

_____

_____

_____

Let the healing begin!

Full body check in

DATE _____

THINGS I LIKE ABOUT MY SKIN
○ _____
○ _____
○ _____

HOW DRY/OILY IS MY SKIN TODAY

(1) (2) (3) (4) (5)
(6) (7) (8) (9) (10)

MARK WHERE YOUR BREAKOUT IS

FRONT   BACK

STRESS/EMOTIONAL LEVEL

HOW DOES YOUR SKIN FEEL TODAY?
○ _____
○ _____
○ _____

TODAY'S MEALS/SNACKS
○ _____
○ _____
○ _____
○ _____
○ _____
○ _____

HOW MANY GLASSES OF WATER DID I HAVE TODAY?

LIST ANY MEDICATIONS(HERBAL OR PRESCRIBED TAKEN FOR SKIN RELIEF)
○ _____
○ _____
○ _____

DAILY SKIN JOURNALING

Day 1

_____

_____

_____

_____

_____

_____

_____

_____

_____

_____

WHAT HAVE I USED ON MY SKIN?

_____

_____

_____

WHAT IS THE GOAL FOR MY SKIN TODAY?

_____

_____

_____

Full body check in

DATE _____

THINGS I LIKE ABOUT MY SKIN _____
- ○ _____
- ○ _____
- ○ _____

HOW DRY/OILY IS MY SKIN TODAY

(1) (2) (3) (4) (5)
(6) (7) (8) (9) (10)

MARK WHERE YOUR BREAKOUT IS

FRONT   BACK

STRESS/EMOTIONAL LEVEL _____

HOW DOES YOUR SKIN FEEL TODAY? _____
- ○ _____
- ○ _____
- ○ _____

TODAY'S MEALS/SNACKS _____
- ○ _____
- ○ _____
- ○ _____
- ○ _____
- ○ _____
- ○ _____

HOW MANY GLASSES OF WATER DID I HAVE TODAY?

LIST ANY MEDICATIONS(HERBAL OR PRESCRIBED TAKEN FOR SKIN RELIEF)
- ○ _____
- ○ _____
- ○ _____

DAILY SKIN JOURNALING

Day 2

_____

_____

_____

_____

_____

_____

_____

_____

_____

_____

_____

_____

WHAT HAVE I USED ON MY SKIN?

_____

_____

_____

WHAT IS THE GOAL FOR MY SKIN TODAY?

_____

_____

_____

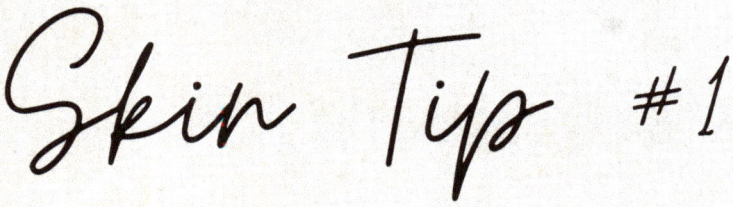

Skin Tip #1

Wash your face with a white cloth, rag, or towelette.

Full body check in

DATE _____

THINGS I LIKE ABOUT MY SKIN
- ○ _____
- ○ _____
- ○ _____

HOW DRY/OILY IS MY SKIN TODAY

1 2 3 4 5
6 7 8 9 10

MARK WHERE YOUR BREAKOUT IS

FRONT   **BACK**

STRESS/EMOTIONAL LEVEL

HOW DOES YOUR SKIN FEEL TODAY? _____
- ○ _____
- ○ _____
- ○ _____

TODAY'S MEALS/SNACKS
- ○ _____
- ○ _____
- ○ _____
- ○ _____
- ○ _____
- ○ _____

HOW MANY GLASSES OF WATER DID I HAVE TODAY?

LIST ANY MEDICATIONS(HERBAL CR PRESCRIBED TAKEN FOR SKIN RELIEF) _____
- ○ _____
- ○ _____
- ○ _____

DAILY SKIN JOURNALING

Day 3

_____

_____

_____

_____

_____

_____

_____

_____

_____

_____

_____

WHAT HAVE I USED ON MY SKIN?

_____

_____

_____

_____

WHAT IS THE GOAL FOR MY SKIN TODAY?

_____

_____

_____

Full body check in

DATE _____

THINGS I LIKE ABOUT MY SKIN
- ○ _____
- ○ _____
- ○ _____

HOW DRY/OILY IS MY SKIN TODAY

① ② ③ ④ ⑤
⑥ ⑦ ⑧ ⑨ ⑩

MARK WHERE YOUR BREAKOUT IS

FRONT　　**BACK**

STRESS/EMOTIONAL LEVEL

HOW DOES YOUR SKIN FEEL TODAY?
- ○ _____
- ○ _____
- ○ _____

TODAY'S MEALS/SNACKS
- ○ _____
- ○ _____
- ○ _____
- ○ _____
- ○ _____
- ○ _____

HOW MANY GLASSES OF WATER DID I HAVE TODAY?

LIST ANY MEDICATIONS(HERBAL OR PRESCRIBED TAKEN FOR SKIN RELIEF)
- ○ _____
- ○ _____
- ○ _____

DAILY SKIN JOURNALING

Day 4

_____

_____

_____

_____

_____

_____

_____

_____

_____

_____

_____

WHAT HAVE I USED ON MY SKIN?

_____

_____

_____

_____

WHAT IS THE GOAL FOR MY SKIN TODAY?

_____

_____

_____

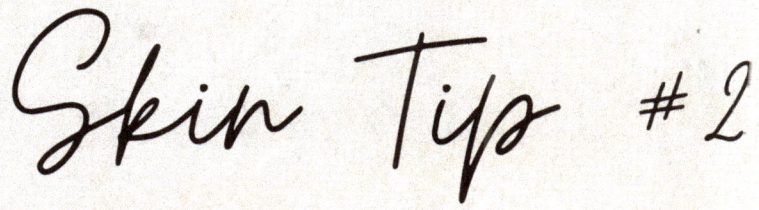

Skin Tip #2

Drink water regularly to keep your skin hydrated.

Full body check in

DATE _____

THINGS I LIKE ABOUT MY SKIN
- ○ _____
- ○ _____
- ○ _____

HOW DRY/OILY IS MY SKIN TODAY

(1) (2) (3) (4) (5)
(6) (7) (8) (9) (10)

MARK WHERE YOUR BREAKOUT IS

FRONT   BACK

STRESS/EMOTIONAL LEVEL

HOW DOES YOUR SKIN FEEL TODAY?
- ○ _____
- ○ _____
- ○ _____

TODAY'S MEALS/SNACKS
- ○ _____
- ○ _____
- ○ _____
- ○ _____
- ○ _____
- ○ _____

HOW MANY GLASSES OF WATER DID I HAVE TODAY?

LIST ANY MEDICATIONS(HERBAL OR PRESCRIBED TAKEN FOR SKIN RELIEF)
- ○ _____
- ○ _____
- ○ _____

DAILY SKIN JOURNALING

Day 5

_____

_____

_____

_____

_____

_____

_____

_____

_____

_____

_____

_____

WHAT HAVE I USED ON MY SKIN?

_____

_____

_____

WHAT IS THE GOAL FOR MY SKIN TODAY?

_____

_____

_____

Full body check in

DATE _____

THINGS I LIKE ABOUT MY SKIN _____
- ○ _____
- ○ _____
- ○ _____

HOW DRY/OILY IS MY SKIN TODAY

1 2 3 4 5
6 7 8 9 10

MARK WHERE YOUR BREAKOUT IS

FRONT   BACK

STRESS/EMOTIONAL LEVEL _____

HOW DOES YOUR SKIN FEEL TODAY? _____
- ○ _____
- ○ _____
- ○ _____

TODAY'S MEALS/SNACKS _____
- ○ _____
- ○ _____
- ○ _____
- ○ _____
- ○ _____
- ○ _____

HOW MANY GLASSES OF WATER DID I HAVE TODAY?

LIST ANY MEDICATIONS(HERBAL OR PRESCRIBED TAKEN FOR SKIN RELIEF)
- ○ _____
- ○ _____
- ○ _____

DAILY SKIN JOURNALING

Day 6

WHAT HAVE I USED ON MY SKIN?

WHAT IS THE GOAL FOR MY SKIN TODAY?

Wash your
clothes and
sheets in a
free & gentle
detergent.

Full body check in

DATE _____

THINGS I LIKE ABOUT MY SKIN
- ○ _____
- ○ _____
- ○ _____

HOW DRY/OILY IS MY SKIN TODAY

(1) (2) (3) (4) (5)
(6) (7) (8) (9) (10)

MARK WHERE YOUR BREAKOUT IS

FRONT   BACK

STRESS/EMOTIONAL LEVEL

HOW DOES YOUR SKIN FEEL TODAY? _____
- ○ _____
- ○ _____
- ○ _____

TODAY'S MEALS/SNACKS _____
- ○ _____
- ○ _____
- ○ _____
- ○ _____
- ○ _____

HOW MANY GLASSES OF WATER DID I HAVE TODAY?

LIST ANY MEDICATIONS(HERBAL OR PRESCRIBED TAKEN FOR SKIN RELIEF)
- ○ _____
- ○ _____
- ○ _____

DAILY SKIN JOURNALING

Day 7

_____

_____

_____

_____

_____

_____

_____

_____

_____

_____

_____

WHAT HAVE I USED ON MY SKIN?

_____

_____

_____

_____

WHAT IS THE GOAL FOR MY SKIN TODAY?

_____

_____

_____

Full body check in

DATE _____

THINGS I LIKE ABOUT MY SKIN _____
○ _____
○ _____
○ _____

HOW DRY/OILY IS MY SKIN TODAY

(1) (2) (3) (4) (5)
(6) (7) (8) (9) (10)

MARK WHERE YOUR BREAKOUT IS

FRONT   BACK

STRESS/EMOTIONAL LEVEL

HOW DOES YOUR SKIN FEEL TODAY? _____
○ _____
○ _____
○ _____

TODAY'S MEALS/SNACKS
○ _____
○ _____
○ _____
○ _____
○ _____
○ _____

HOW MANY GLASSES OF WATER DID I HAVE TODAY?

LIST ANY MEDICATIONS(HERBAL OR PRESCRIBED TAKEN FOR SKIN RELIEF) ___
○ _____
○ _____
○ _____

DAILY SKIN JOURNALING

Day 8

_____

_____

_____

_____

_____

_____

_____

_____

_____

_____

WHAT HAVE I USED ON MY SKIN?

_____

_____

_____

_____

WHAT IS THE GOAL FOR MY SKIN TODAY?

_____

_____

_____

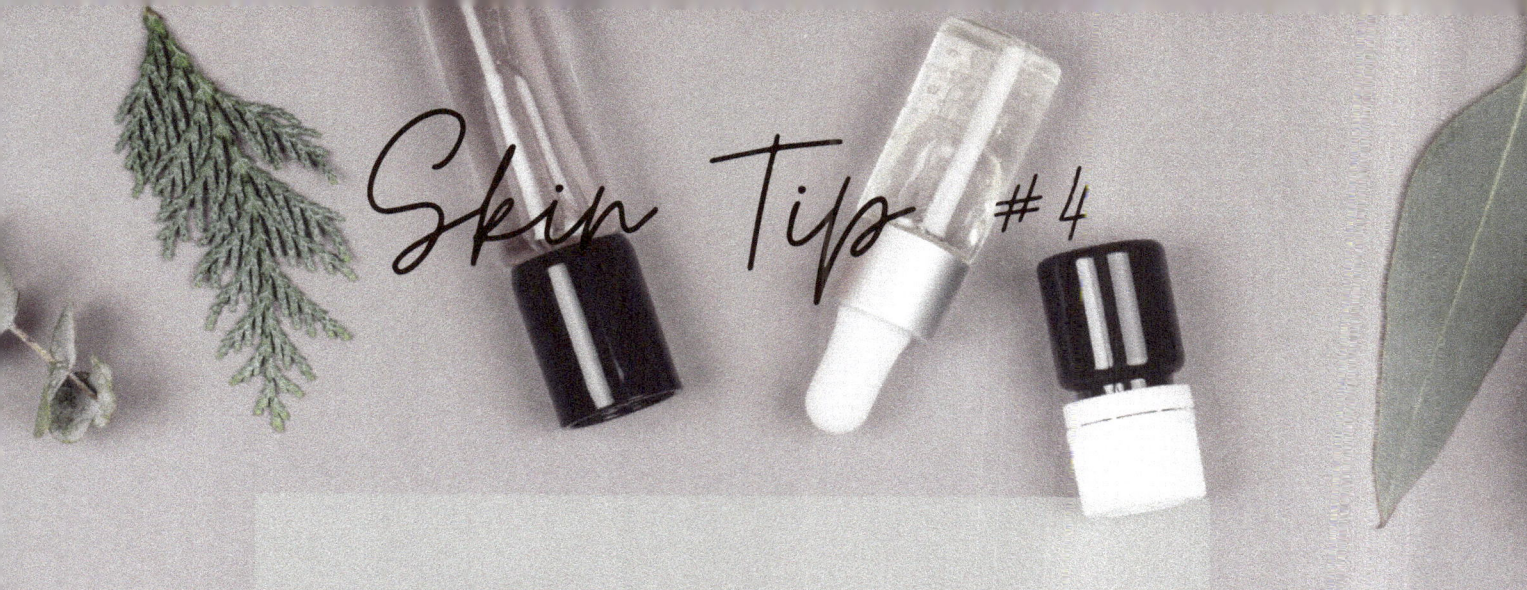

Skin Tip #4

Wash your face and body with warm water instead of hot water.

Full body check in

DATE _____

THINGS I LIKE ABOUT MY SKIN _____
- ○ _____
- ○ _____
- ○ _____

HOW DRY/OILY IS MY SKIN TODAY

1 2 3 4 5
6 7 8 9 10

MARK WHERE YOUR BREAKOUT IS

FRONT   BACK

STRESS/EMOTIONAL LEVEL

HOW DOES YOUR SKIN FEEL TODAY? _____
- ○ _____
- ○ _____
- ○ _____

TODAY'S MEALS/SNACKS _____
- ○ _____
- ○ _____
- ○ _____
- ○ _____
- ○

HOW MANY GLASSES OF WATER DID I HAVE TODAY?

LIST ANY MEDICATIONS(HERBAL OR PRESCRIBED TAKEN FOR SKIN RELIEF) _____
- ○ _____
- ○ _____
- ○ _____

DAILY SKIN JOURNALING

Day 9

_____

_____

_____

_____

_____

_____

_____

_____

_____

_____

_____

WHAT HAVE I USED ON MY SKIN?

_____

_____

_____

WHAT IS THE GOAL FOR MY SKIN TODAY?

_____

_____

_____

Full body check in

DATE _____

THINGS I LIKE ABOUT MY SKIN
○ _____
○ _____
○ _____

HOW DRY/OILY IS MY SKIN TODAY

(1) (2) (3) (4) (5)
(6) (7) (8) (9) (10)

MARK WHERE YOUR BREAKOUT IS

FRONT   BACK

STRESS/EMOTIONAL LEVEL

HOW DOES YOUR SKIN FEEL TODAY?
○ _____
○ _____
○ _____

TODAY'S MEALS/SNACKS
○ _____
○ _____
○ _____
○ _____
○ _____
○ _____

HOW MANY GLASSES OF WATER DID I HAVE TODAY?

LIST ANY MEDICATIONS(HERBAL OR PRESCRIBED TAKEN FOR SKIN RELIEF)
○ _____
○ _____
○ _____

DAILY SKIN JOURNALING

Day 10

_____

_____

_____

_____

_____

_____

_____

_____

_____

_____

_____

WHAT HAVE I USED ON MY SKIN?

_____

_____

_____

WHAT IS THE GOAL FOR MY SKIN TODAY?

_____

_____

_____

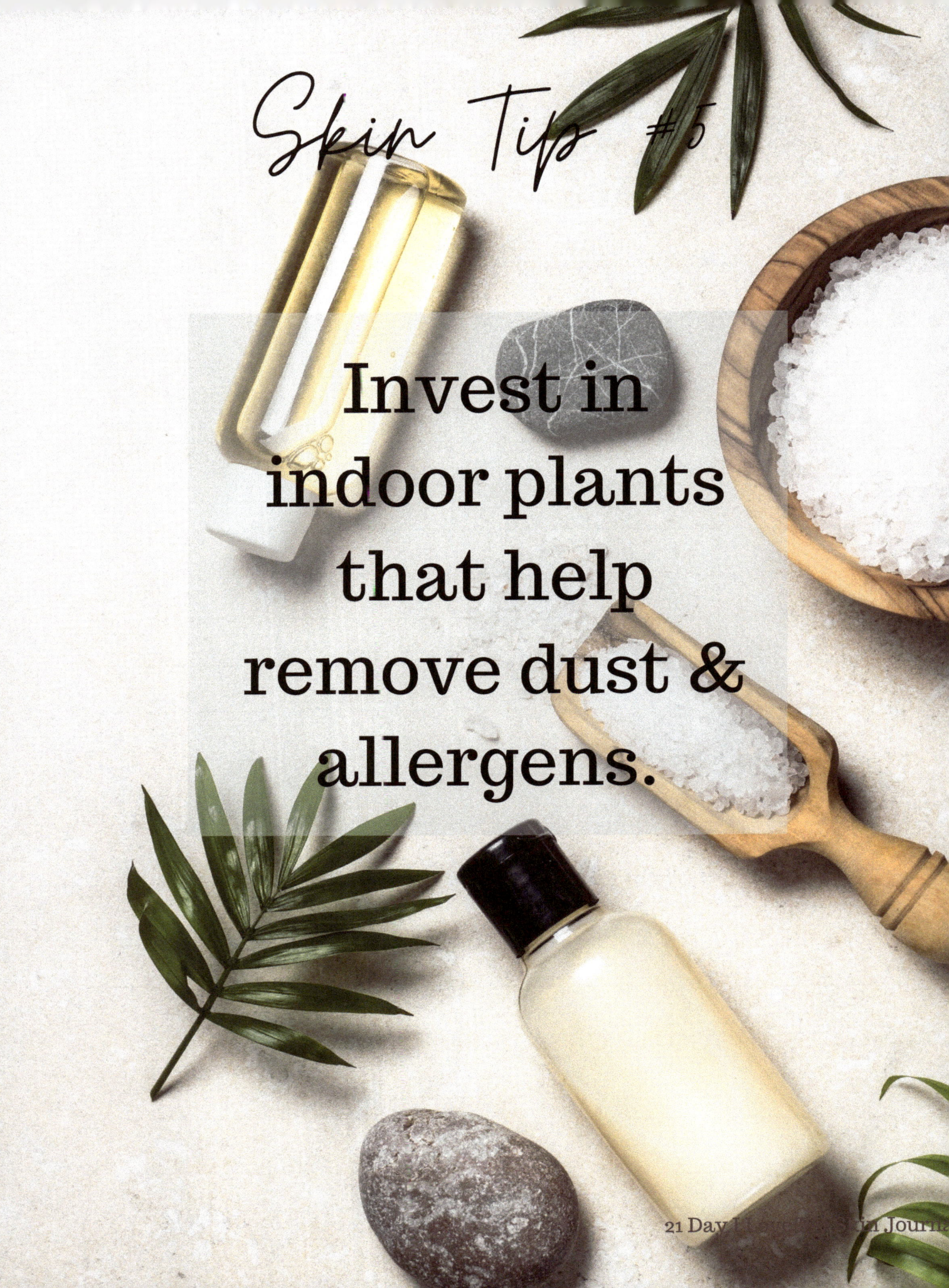

Skin Tip #5

Invest in indoor plants that help remove dust & allergens.

Full body check in

DATE _____

THINGS I LIKE ABOUT MY SKIN
○ _____
○ _____
○ _____

HOW DRY/OILY IS MY SKIN TODAY

(1) (2) (3) (4) (5)
(6) (7) (8) (9) (10)

MARK WHERE YOUR BREAKOUT IS

FRONT   **BACK**

STRESS/EMOTIONAL LEVEL

HOW DOES YOUR SKIN FEEL TODAY? _____
○ _____
○ _____
○ _____

TODAY'S MEALS/SNACKS _____
○ _____
○ _____
○ _____
○ _____
○ _____
○ _____

HOW MANY GLASSES OF WATER DID I HAVE TODAY?

LIST ANY MEDICATIONS(HERBAL OR PRESCRIBED TAKEN FOR SKIN RELIEF
○ _____
○ _____
○ _____

DAILY SKIN JOURNALING

Day 11

WHAT HAVE I USED ON MY SKIN?

WHAT IS THE GOAL FOR MY SKIN TODAY?

Full body check in

DATE _____

THINGS I LIKE ABOUT MY SKIN _____
- ○ _____
- ○ _____
- ○ _____

HOW DRY/OILY IS MY SKIN TODAY

① ② ③ ④ ⑤
⑥ ⑦ ⑧ ⑨ ⑩

MARK WHERE YOUR BREAKOUT IS

FRONT   BACK

STRESS/EMOTIONAL LEVEL _____

HOW DOES YOUR SKIN FEEL TODAY? _____
- ○ _____
- ○ _____
- ○ _____

TODAY'S MEALS/SNACKS _____
- ○ _____
- ○ _____
- ○ _____
- ○ _____
- ○ _____

HOW MANY GLASSES OF WATER DID I HAVE TODAY?

LIST ANY MEDICATIONS(HERBAL OF PRESCRIBED TAKEN FOR SKIN RELIEF) _____
- ○ _____
- ○ _____
- ○ _____

DAILY SKIN JOURNALING

Day 12

_____

_____

_____

_____

_____

_____

_____

_____

_____

_____

_____

WHAT HAVE I USED ON MY SKIN?

_____

_____

_____

_____

WHAT IS THE GOAL FOR MY SKIN TODAY?

_____

_____

_____

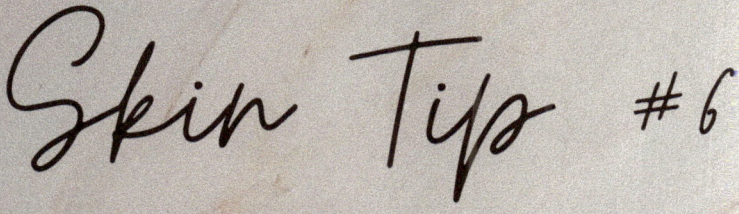

Skin Tip #6

Limit your intake of dairy products.

Full body check in

DATE _____

HOW DOES YOUR SKIN FEEL TODAY?
- ○ _____
- ○ _____
- ○ _____

THINGS I LIKE ABOUT MY SKIN
- ○ _____
- ○ _____
- ○ _____

TODAY'S MEALS/SNACKS
- ○ _____
- ○ _____
- ○ _____
- ○ _____
- ○ _____
- ○ _____

HOW DRY/OILY IS MY SKIN TODAY

1 2 3 4 5
6 7 8 9 10

MARK WHERE YOUR BREAKOUT IS

FRONT   BACK

HOW MANY GLASSES OF WATER DID I HAVE TODAY?

LIST ANY MEDICATIONS(HERBAL OR PRESCRIBED TAKEN FOR SKIN RELIEF)
- ○ _____
- ○ _____
- ○ _____

STRESS/EMOTIONAL LEVEL

DAILY SKIN JOURNALING

Day 13

_____

_____

_____

_____

_____

_____

_____

_____

_____

WHAT HAVE I USED ON MY SKIN?

_____

_____

_____

WHAT IS THE GOAL FOR MY SKIN TODAY?

_____

_____

Full body check in

DATE _____

THINGS I LIKE ABOUT MY SKIN _____
- ○ _____
- ○ _____
- ○ _____

HOW DRY/OILY IS MY SKIN TODAY

(1) (2) (3) (4) (5)
(6) (7) (8) (9) (10)

MARK WHERE YOUR BREAKOUT IS

FRONT   BACK

STRESS/EMOTIONAL LEVEL

HOW DOES YOUR SKIN FEEL TODAY? _____
- ○ _____
- ○ _____
- ○ _____

TODAY'S MEALS/SNACKS _____
- ○ _____
- ○ _____
- ○ _____
- ○ _____
- ○ _____
- ○ _____

HOW MANY GLASSES OF WATER DID I HAVE TODAY?

LIST ANY MEDICATIONS(HERBAL OR PRESCRIBED TAKEN FOR SKIN RELIEF)
- ○ _____
- ○ _____
- ○ _____

DAILY SKIN JOURNALING

Day 14

_____
_____
_____
_____
_____
_____
_____
_____
_____
_____
_____

WHAT HAVE I USED ON MY SKIN?

_____
_____
_____
_____

WHAT IS THE GOAL FOR MY SKIN TODAY?

_____
_____
_____

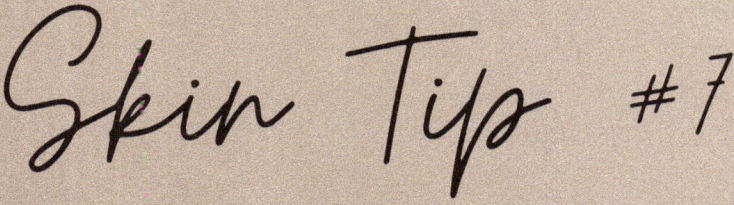

Skin Tip #7

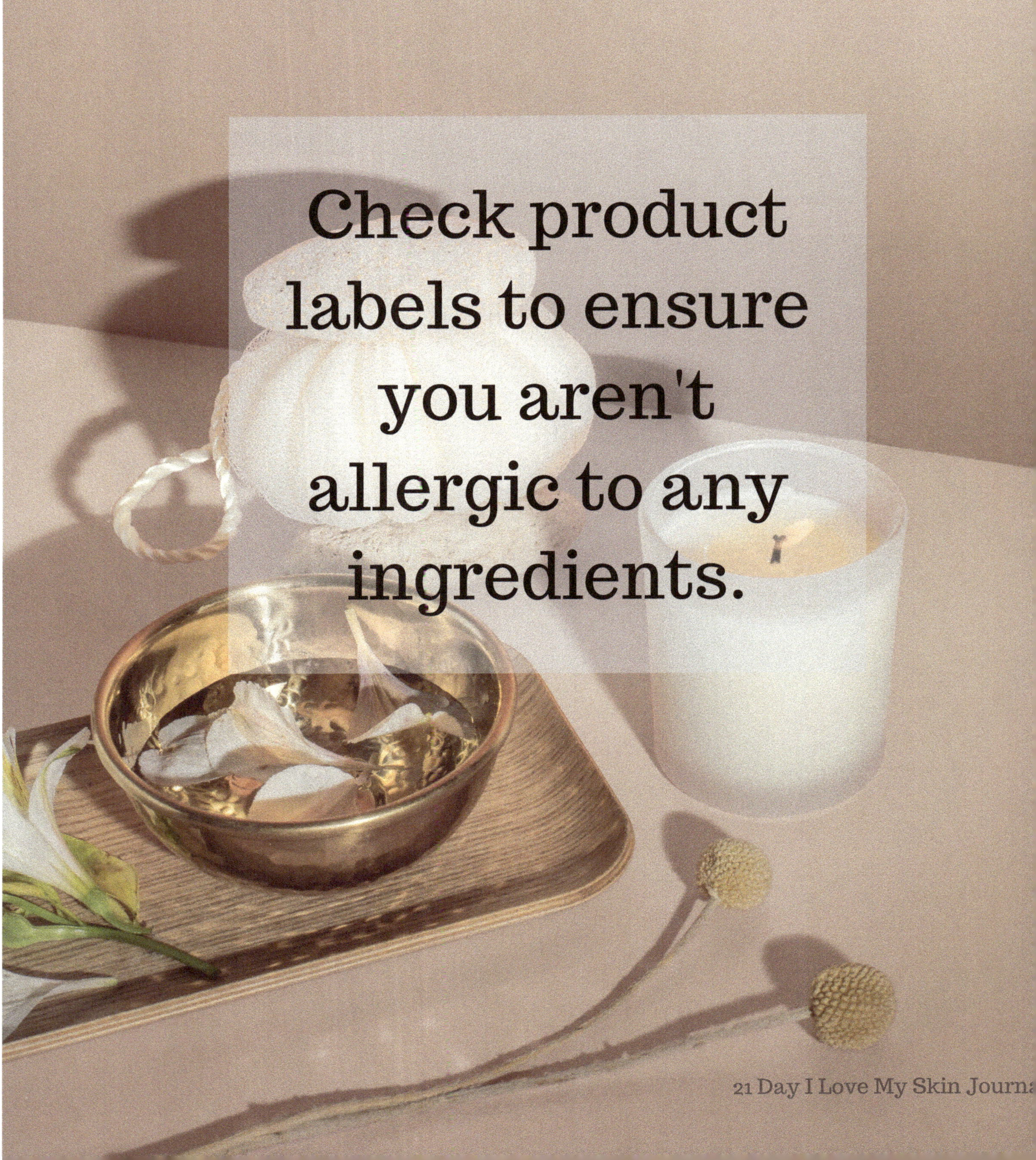

Check product labels to ensure you aren't allergic to any ingredients.

Full body check in

DATE _____

THINGS I LIKE ABOUT MY SKIN
- ○ _____
- ○ _____
- ○ _____

HOW DRY/OILY IS MY SKIN TODAY

① ② ③ ④ ⑤
⑥ ⑦ ⑧ ⑨ ⑩

MARK WHERE YOUR BREAKOUT IS

FRONT   BACK

STRESS/EMOTIONAL LEVEL

HOW DOES YOUR SKIN FEEL TODAY? _____
- ○ _____
- ○ _____
- ○ _____

TODAY'S MEALS/SNACKS _____
- ○ _____
- ○ _____
- ○ _____
- ○ _____
- ○ _____

HOW MANY GLASSES OF WATER DID I HAVE TODAY?

LIST ANY MEDICATIONS(HERBAL OR PRESCRIBED TAKEN FOR SKIN RELIEF)
- ○ _____
- ○ _____
- ○ _____

DAILY SKIN JOURNALING

Day 15

_____

_____

_____

_____

_____

_____

_____

_____

_____

_____

_____

WHAT HAVE I USED ON MY SKIN?

_____

_____

_____

_____

WHAT IS THE GOAL FOR MY SKIN TODAY?

_____

_____

_____

Full body check in

DATE _____

HOW DOES YOUR SKIN FEEL TODAY? _____
- ○ _____
- ○ _____
- ○ _____

THINGS I LIKE ABOUT MY SKIN
- ○ _____
- ○ _____
- ○ _____

TODAY'S MEALS/SNACKS
- ○ _____
- ○ _____
- ○ _____
- ○ _____
- ○ _____
- ○ _____

HOW DRY/OILY IS MY SKIN TODAY

1 2 3 4 5
6 7 8 9 10

MARK WHERE YOUR BREAKOUT IS

FRONT   BACK

HOW MANY GLASSES OF WATER DID I HAVE TODAY?

LIST ANY MEDICATIONS(HERBAL OR PRESCRIBED TAKEN FOR SKIN RELIEF)
- ○ _____
- ○ _____
- ○ _____

STRESS/EMOTIONAL LEVEL

DAILY SKIN JOURNALING

Day 16

_____

_____

_____

_____

_____

_____

_____

_____

_____

_____

WHAT HAVE I USED ON MY SKIN?

_____

_____

_____

_____

WHAT IS THE GOAL FOR MY SKIN TODAY?

_____

_____

_____

Skin Tip #8

Do not over exfoliate. It causes your skin barrier to break, resulting in breakouts, dry skin, etc.

Full body check in

DATE _____

THINGS I LIKE ABOUT MY SKIN
- ○ _____
- ○ _____
- ○ _____

HOW DRY/OILY IS MY SKIN TODAY

① ② ③ ④ ⑤
⑥ ⑦ ⑧ ⑨ ⑩

MARK WHERE YOUR BREAKOUT IS

FRONT   BACK

STRESS/EMOTIONAL LEVEL

HOW DOES YOUR SKIN FEEL TODAY?
- ○ _____
- ○ _____
- ○ _____

TODAY'S MEALS/SNACKS
- ○ _____
- ○ _____
- ○ _____
- ○ _____
- ○ _____
- ○ _____

HOW MANY GLASSES OF WATER DID I HAVE TODAY?

LIST ANY MEDICATIONS(HERBAL OR PRESCRIBED TAKEN FOR SKIN RELIEF)
- ○ _____
- ○ _____
- ○ _____

DAILY SKIN JOURNALING

Day 17

_____

_____

_____

_____

_____

_____

_____

_____

_____

_____

_____

WHAT HAVE I USED ON MY SKIN?

_____

_____

_____

WHAT IS THE GOAL FOR MY SKIN TODAY?

_____

_____

_____

Full body check in

DATE _____

THINGS I LIKE ABOUT MY SKIN _____
- ○ _____
- ○ _____
- ○ _____

HOW DRY/OILY IS MY SKIN TODAY

① ② ③ ④ ⑤
⑥ ⑦ ⑧ ⑨ ⑩

MARK WHERE YOUR BREAKOUT IS

FRONT   BACK

STRESS/EMOTIONAL LEVEL

HOW DOES YOUR SKIN FEEL TODAY?
- ○ _____
- ○ _____
- ○ _____

TODAY'S MEALS/SNACKS
- ○ _____
- ○ _____
- ○ _____
- ○ _____
- ○ _____
- ○ _____

HOW MANY GLASSES OF WATER DID I HAVE TODAY?

LIST ANY MEDICATIONS(HERBAL OR PRESCRIBED TAKEN FOR SKIN RELIEF)
- ○ _____
- ○ _____
- ○ _____

DAILY SKIN JOURNALING

Day 1

_____

_____

_____

_____

_____

_____

_____

_____

_____

_____

_____

WHAT HAVE I USED ON MY SKIN?

_____

_____

_____

WHAT IS THE GOAL FOR MY SKIN TODAY?

_____

_____

_____

Skin Tip #9

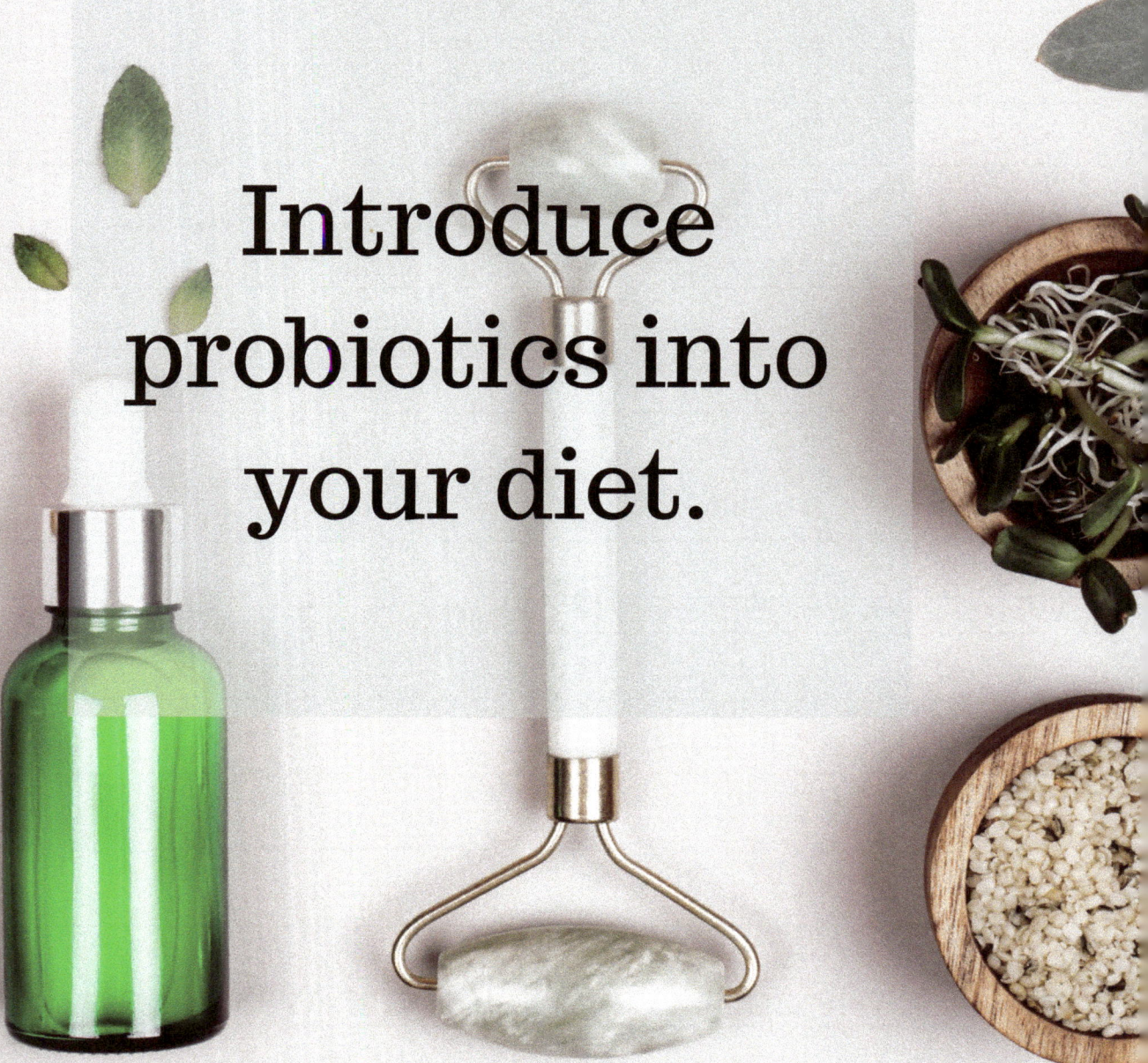

Introduce probiotics into your diet.

Full body check in

DATE _____

THINGS I LIKE ABOUT MY SKIN
- ○ _____
- ○ _____
- ○ _____

HOW DRY/OILY IS MY SKIN TODAY

(1) (2) (3) (4) (5)
(6) (7) (8) (9) (10)

MARK WHERE YOUR BREAKOUT IS

FRONT   BACK

STRESS/EMOTIONAL LEVEL

HOW DOES YOUR SKIN FEEL TODAY?
- ○ _____
- ○ _____
- ○ _____

TODAY'S MEALS/SNACKS
- ○ _____
- ○ _____
- ○ _____
- ○ _____
- ○ _____
- ○ _____

HOW MANY GLASSES OF WATER DID I HAVE TODAY?

LIST ANY MEDICATIONS(HERBAL OR PRESCRIBED TAKEN FOR SKIN RELIEF)
- ○ _____
- ○ _____
- ○ _____

DAILY SKIN JOURNALING

Day 19

_____

_____

_____

_____

_____

_____

_____

_____

_____

_____

_____

_____

WHAT HAVE I USED ON MY SKIN?

_____

_____

_____

_____

WHAT IS THE GOAL FOR MY SKIN TODAY?

_____

_____

_____

Full body check in

DATE _____

THINGS I LIKE ABOUT MY SKIN
- ○ _____
- ○ _____
- ○ _____

HOW DRY/OILY IS MY SKIN TODAY

(1) (2) (3) (4) (5)
(6) (7) (8) (9) (10)

MARK WHERE YOUR BREAKOUT IS

FRONT   BACK

STRESS/EMOTIONAL LEVEL

HOW DOES YOUR SKIN FEEL TODAY?
- ○ _____
- ○ _____
- ○ _____

TODAY'S MEALS/SNACKS
- ○ _____
- ○ _____
- ○ _____
- ○ _____
- ○ _____
- ○ _____

HOW MANY GLASSES OF WATER DID I HAVE TODAY?

LIST ANY MEDICATIONS(HERBAL OR PRESCRIBED TAKEN FOR SKIN RELIEF)
- ○ _____
- ○ _____
- ○ _____

DAILY SKIN JOURNALING

Day 20

_____

_____

_____

_____

_____

_____

_____

_____

_____

_____

_____

WHAT HAVE I USED ON MY SKIN?

_____

_____

_____

_____

WHAT IS THE GOAL FOR MY SKIN TODAY?

_____

_____

_____

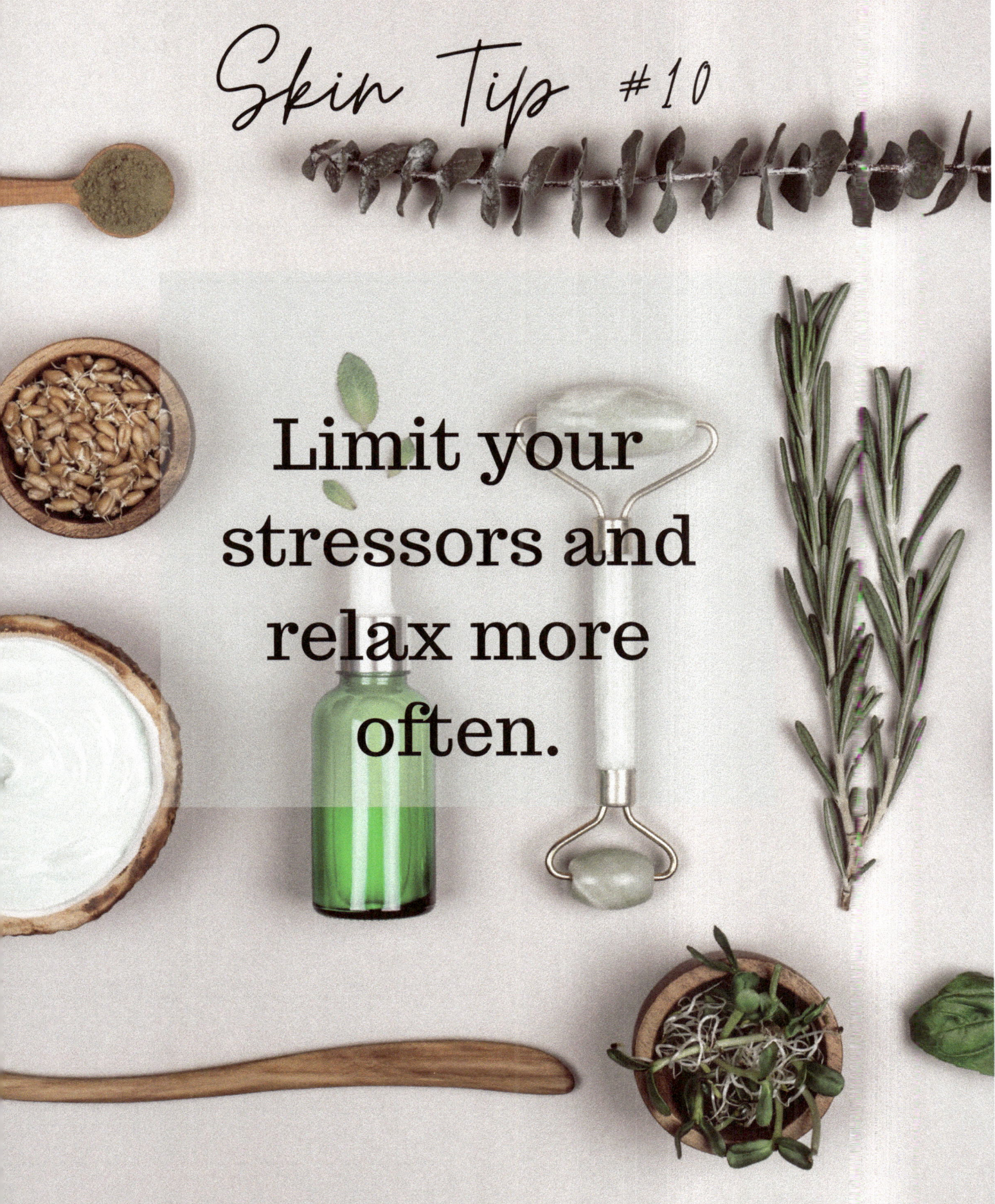

Skin Tip #10

Limit your stressors and relax more often.

Full body check in

DATE _____

THINGS I LIKE ABOUT MY SKIN

○ _____

○ _____

○ _____

HOW DRY/OILY IS MY SKIN TODAY

1 2 3 4 5

6 7 8 9 10

MARK WHERE YOUR BREAKOUT IS

FRONT   BACK

STRESS/EMOTIONAL LEVEL

HOW DOES YOUR SKIN FEEL TODAY?

○ _____

○ _____

○ _____

TODAY'S MEALS/SNACKS

○ _____

○ _____

○ _____

○ _____

○ _____

○ _____

HOW MANY GLASSES OF WATER DID I HAVE TODAY?

LIST ANY MEDICATIONS(HERBAL OR PRESCRIBED TAKEN FOR SKIN RELIEF)

○ _____

○ _____

○ _____

DAILY SKIN JOURNALING

Day 21

_____

_____

_____

_____

_____

_____

_____

_____

_____

_____

WHAT HAVE I USED ON MY SKIN?

_____

_____

_____

WHAT IS THE GOAL FOR MY SKIN TODAY?

_____

_____

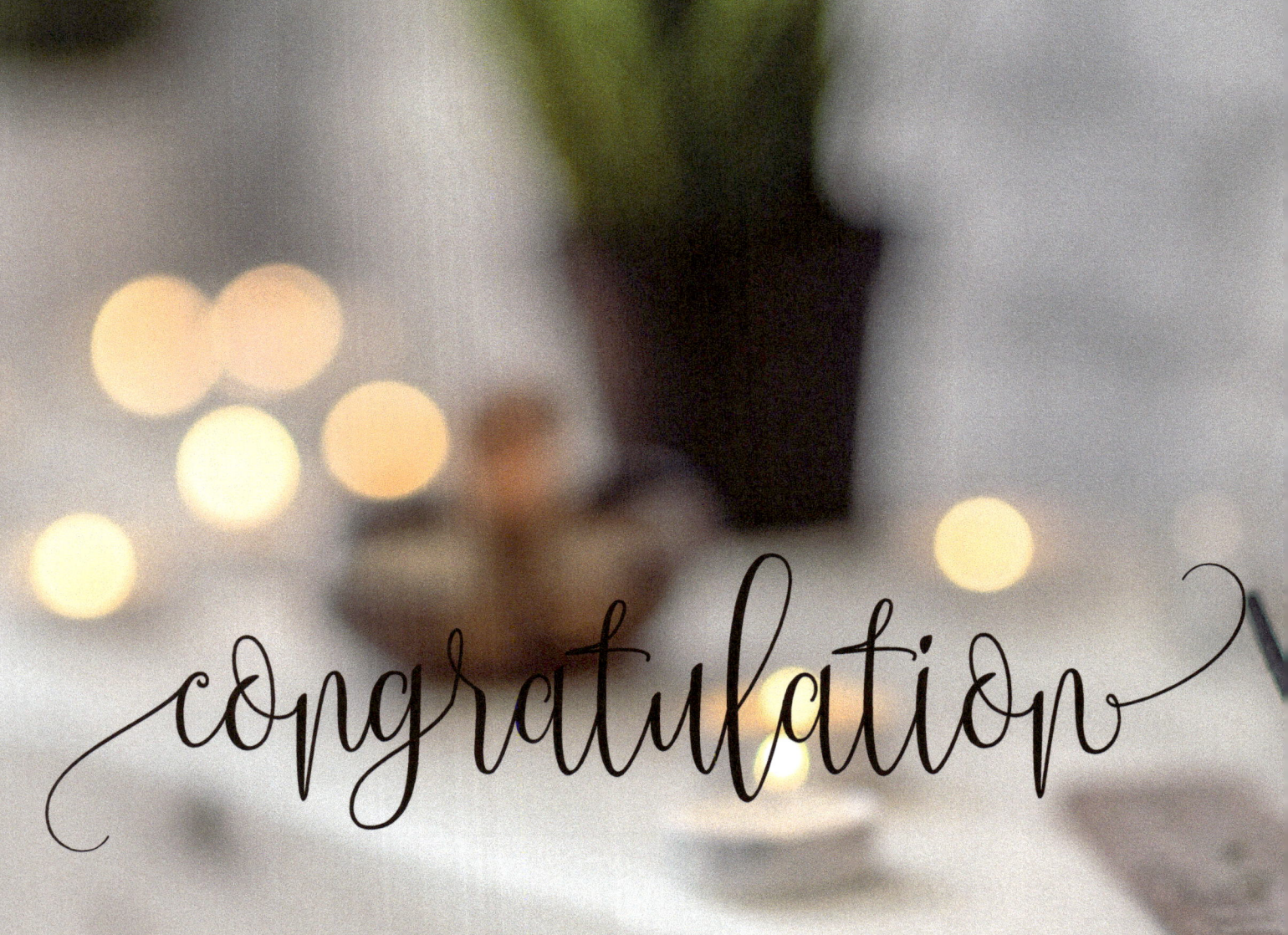

congratulation

You've completed your 21 Day Skin Loving Journey! I am proud of you for completing this journey and taking the steps to love every part of your skin! DON'T STOP LOVING ALL OF YOU!

~Empress

Now that you have completed the 21-Day Journey, write a letter to yourself about how this has helped, what you have learned to love about yourself, and how you much you appreciate about this journey.

Dear _____

_____

_____

_____

_____

_____

_____

_____

_____

_____

_____

_____